OMGhee

Your Guide to making Ghee at home

Spencer Ash

A catalog record for this book is available.

ISBN-13: 978-1482070484
ISBN-10: 1482070480

The information included in this book is for educational purposes only. It is not intended to be a substitute for professional medical advice.

Table of Contents

What is Ghee?

Ghee is a type of clarified butter that is prepared by melting un-salted (and preferably grass-fed) butter until the water evaporates and the milk solids in the butter separate and settle on the bottom of the pan. Although ghee is a form of clarified butter, they are not one in the same: ghee is cooked longer and the butterfats are browned giving the finished product a nutty flavor.

The proteins and caseins found in milk solids can have negative health effects, which we will get later. In the process of making ghee, the milk solids are rendered from the butter and are then filtered out leaving pure, delicious, and healthy butter fat that is perfect for cooking. After the milk solids have been removed, there is also no longer a need for refrigeration (ghee can be kept in a sealed jar for several months)!

In Indian cultures, ghee is a sacred food and is believed to have many health promoting properties and is central to the Ayurveda, a 5,000 year old system of traditional medicine. Pure ghee, in addition to being a concentrated source of nutrition is believed to contain healing properties and is often eaten on its own or with herbs and spices. Ghee is also regarded by the Ayurveda to be a rasayana, or a source containing rejuvenating properties that can reduce inflammation with its cooling energies. Because of these properties, ghee is commonly applied to small wounds, cuts, and burns to increase healing.

Ghee: delicious, healthy, awesome.

Butter vs. Ghee

(and why Ghee wins!)

Butter is a concentrated solid-fat dairy product that is made by churning the cream or milk of animals such as cows, goats, and sheep. Most butter is comprised of about 80% fat (good saturated fats) and the rest is made up of water and milk solids (proteins and salts).

In almost all dairy products (butter included) dairy proteins, such as casein and whey, are found. These proteins can negatively effect a persons health as they contain both growth and immune factors also known as hormones. In addition dairy products, because they contain specific "milk solids" can provoke inflammatory responses in the gut that adversely affect the digestion of food, spike insulin levels, and even have an acidifying effect on the body (all potentially bad stuff). The proteins contained in butter are no different than other dairy proteins and may contribute to certain conditions such as: autoimmune disease, cancer, and cardiovascular disease.

The take away: the dairy proteins contained in that milk solids found in butter are *bad*.

With ghee, *there are no milk solids or bad dairy proteins*...they have been filtered out during the clarification process (thats *good* news)! There are no major downsides to consuming butter once it goes through this process. The clarification process in making ghee removes the milk proteins (and salts) from the butter and leaves behind pure, golden butterfat. *Remember, clarified butter and ghee are similar but they are not the same, there are a few additional steps required to make ghee.

The Health Benefits of Ghee

Ghee is a pure, clarified butter. As such, it contains no artificial add tives, preservatives, salts, trans fats, or hydrogenated oils. In making ghee from butter a l milk solids are removed during the rendering process making ghee a healthy alternative that is free of problematic milk proteins and suitable for those with dairy sensitiv ties.

Nutrient Absorption:

One of the main benefits associated with ghee is its ability to aid in nutrient absorption within the body. When consumed, ghee easily bonds with lipid-soluble nutrients in food that then may be absorbed by the body's cell walls. This is the reason that ghee is used as a ghrita in the Ayurveda, as it helps to enhance the benefits of certain herbs by allowing the beneficial components to become absorbed into the bodies' cells. Ghee is also a rich source of antioxidants and helps the body to absorb vitamins and minerals from other foods, thus increasing the amount of nutrition that is provided to muscles, tissues, and other systems. Ghee also contains a high concentration of butanoic acid (a fatty acid that can be found in butter) that has anti-bacterial and anti-cancer properties.

Inflammation:

Ayurveda medicine has traditionally used ghee in place of butter for its various healing benefits. One benefit of the benefits of incorporating ghee into the diet are the incredible anti-inflammatory properties that it contains. Ghee is able to naturally lubricate connective tissues in the body, helping to improve flexibility and the bodies' absorption of antioxidants. In Ayurveda medicine, ghee is often used for the treatment of cuts, blisters, burns and also as a remedy for improving the general health of a persons skin.

Digestive Health:

Evidence suggests that ghee may also be a powerful agent for digestive health. When used in the place of butters, oils and other fats, ghee may be able to help reduce stomach acid by protecting and repairing the stomach lining. The same effects that ghee has as a healing agent for cuts, burns, and blisters also make it effective for treating discomfort caused by toxins and acids that build up in the digestive system; as it stimulates the secretion of stomach acids that aid in digestion (butter and other oils achieve the opposite affect).

Making the Ghee

Get ready to make some awesome buttery goodness!

The Materials:

1 Cup unsalted grass-fed butter	1 Medium Skillet (preferably cast iron)	Cheesecloth or Coffee Filter (multiple layers)
1 Rubberband	1 Jar	About 10 minutes

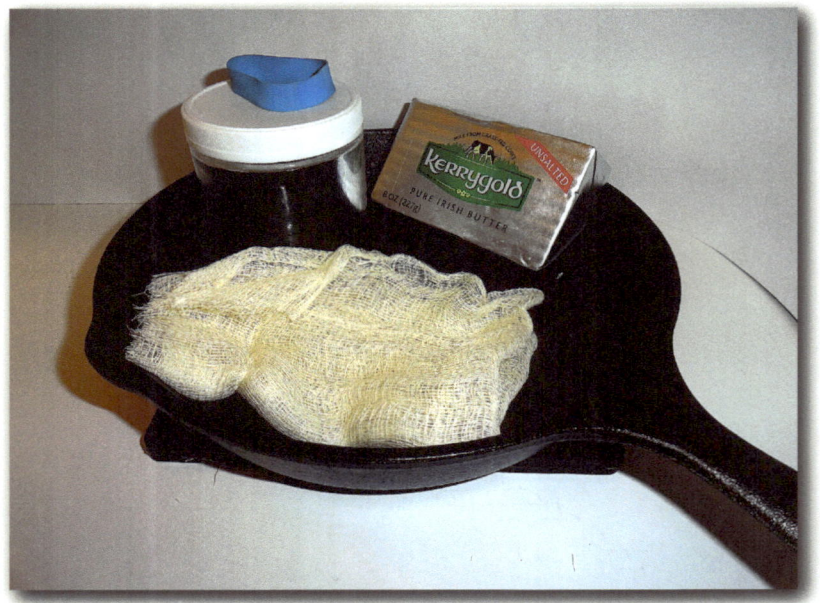

The Preparation:

Begin with 1 cup of unsalted butter (preferably from grass fed cows). Remember that you are making ghee because you care about your health, don't skimp on the butter - quality matters (we suggest using Kerrygold unsalted grassfed butter).

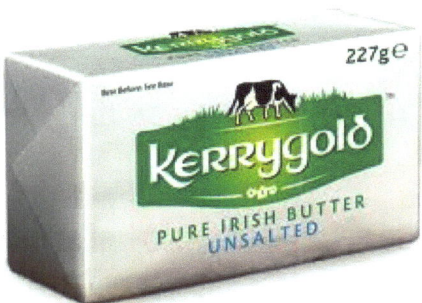

When selecting the butter that you are going to be using remember that you are making ghee because you care about your health. Quality matters so try to take the following into account when selecting your butter:

• *Grass-fed or pastured:*

The cows that produced your butter must be grass-fed, or pastured. This means that they were raised on natural diets, the largest contributing factor affecting the overall health of the cow and thus the milk it produces. Pastured / Grass fed cows are allowed to roam free eating their natural diet and are treated in a humane fashion. Cows raised in this manner are typically happier and healthier and produce higher quality milk, which leads to higher quality and healthy butter.

• *Organic:*

The cows that produced your butter must not have been given hormones or antibiotics. They also must not have been exposed to synthetic pesticides or any other banned chemical substances. The less "junk" that is in the cow's environment means less of bad stuff in your butter.

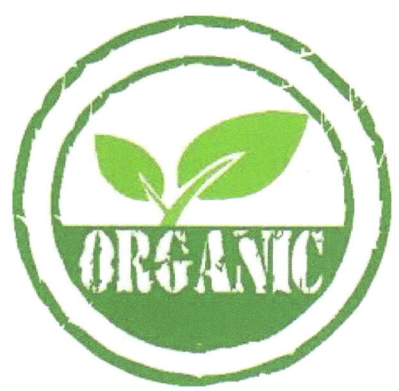

The Process:

Step 1 - Begin heating your skillet (make sure that it is clean and dry).

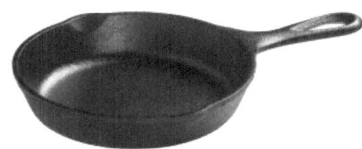

We recommend using a *cast iron skillet* for the following reasons:

- *Cooking in Cast Iron Makes Food Tastes Great:*
  Cast iron distributes heat evenly over the cooking surface, second only to copper pans. This is extremely important when it comes to rendering the milk solids in your butter.

- *Cooking in Cast Iron Is Healthy:*
  First, cast iron pans are a great way to get trace amounts of iron into your diet. Then there is the question raised about the dangers of cooking surfaces such as the teflon that is often found in cookware (cast iron has none).

- *Cooking in Cast Iron is Versatile:*
  Today, cast iron can be found in use from all sorts of people--from the gourmet chef to the campfire cook.

- *Cooking in Cast Iron Is Responsible:*
  When treated well (and often even when not!) cast iron can last for generations - Cast Iron is extremely durable and will last for ever if you take care of it.

Step 2 - Place your butter into your heated skillet and over low heat melt it.

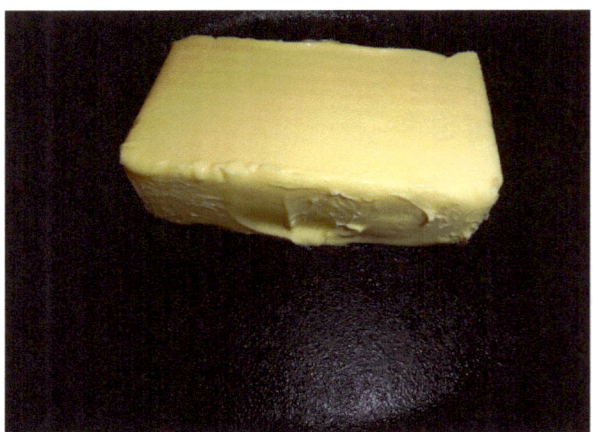

Step 3 - Allow the butter to melt completely. You will begin to see the clear butter fat separate from the milk solids and the butter should be bubbling slightly. The bubbling of the butter signals that the water is beginning to be cooked off, you should hear a crackling noise.

Step 4 - Reduce the heat and wait for the bubbles to get smaller. Eventually they will begin to resemble a foam. Your milk solids should begin to brown shortly after the foam has formed.

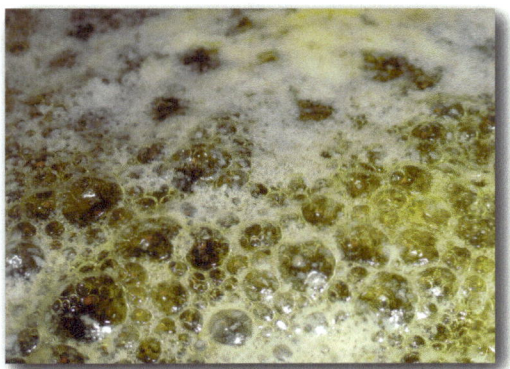

Once the milk solids have turned a golden brown color and begin to sink to the bottom it will be time to remove your skillet from the heating element (approximately 10 minutes after the butter began to bubble).

Your ghee is done when the crackling subsides and the ghee becomes a clear golden yellow with milk solids settling on the bottom of the pan. You may also cook the ghee longer - this will burn the milk solids giving the ghee a darker color and a nuttier flavor almost that of hazelnuts.

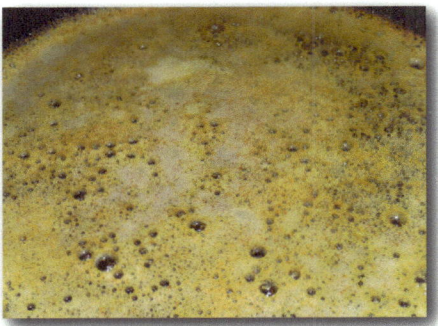

Step 5 - Fold your cheesecloth or coffee filter into multiple layers and secure it to your jar with the rubber band.

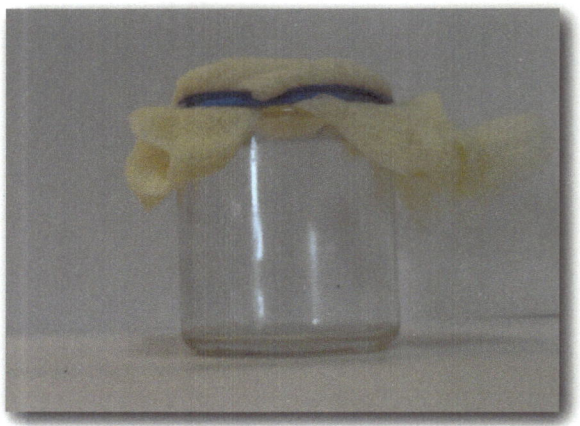

Step 6 - Pour the hot ghee the skillet into the cheesecloth (you may also pour the ghee from the pan into a heat-safe measuring cup and then into the jar to make the pouring easier). Once you have Poured you filtered ghee into your storage jar discard the cheesecloth that is full of toasted milk solids.

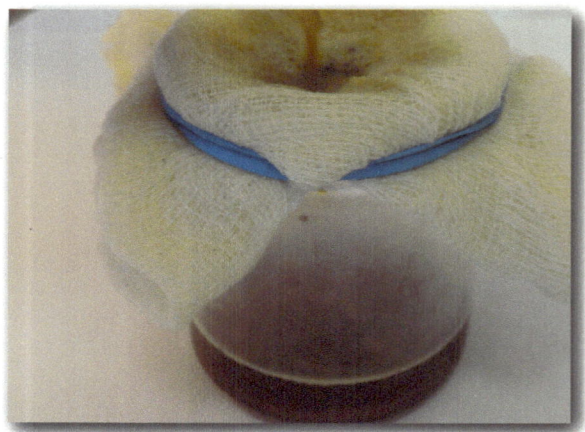

Step 7 - Store your ghee in your sealed jar. Although it is not necessary to refrigerate your ghee since all of the milk solids have been removed, toss it in the fridge to be on the safe side.

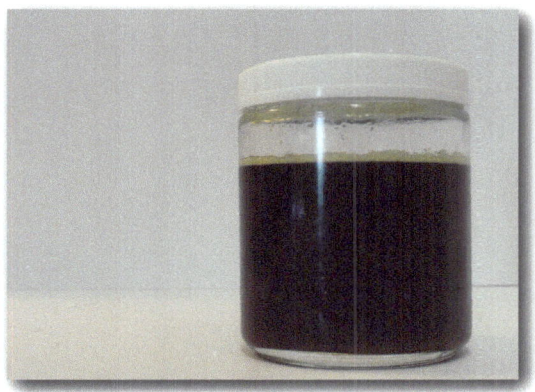

Step 8 - Your will solidify into a solid form once the heat from cooking dissipates.

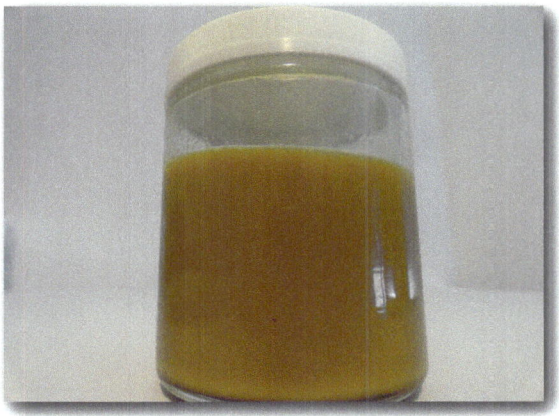

Step 9 - Enjoy your homemade ghee! Check out some of the suggestions in the next section.

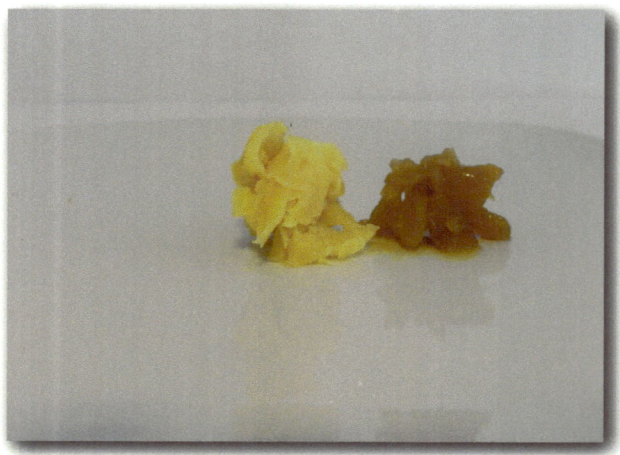

How to Use Your Ghee:

Breakfast:

- Scramble or fry eggs in ghee – they won't stick to the pan.
- Make a French-style omelet with ghee; it's firm and won't turn brown like with butter.
- Use to sauté bacon; works great, tastes great, and won't stick to the pan.
- Sauté veggies such as onion, tomato, and mushrooms in ghee; whisk in beaten eggs and make a breakfast frittata.

Main courses and Soups:

- Stir into piping hot soup just before serving.
- Drizzle over fish, lobster, scallops, or crab.
- Combine minced garlic with plenty of dried herbs such as thyme, rosemary, sage, and parsley. Add salt, pepper, and enough ghee to make an herb paste; rub into a chicken and roast until done – be sure to baste with pan juices!
- Vegetable, Potato, and Dishes
- Drizzle over fresh steamed veggies.

Stir fry greens such as kale, collards, and Swiss chard in ghee for great flavor and digestibility.

- Coat root vegetables with ghee, salt, and pepper; cover and roast at 425 °F until tender.
- Ideal for sautéing or caramelizing onions.
- Spread onto hot sweet potato, or stir into hot mashed sweet potatoes.
- Rub ghee into the skins of sweet potatoes; prick with a fork and bake at 400 °F until tender. Sauté mushrooms in ghee with a splash of wine and a pinch of salt for the best mushrooms ever!

Desserts:

- Use in cakes and cookies; they'll taste great and keep fresh longer.
- Melt chocolate; add a spoonful of ghee and enough powdered sugar to make a glaze.
- Use for cakes, quick breads or cookies.
- Stir a tsp into hot pudding before cooling.
- Sauté sliced apples or pears in ghee; sprinkle on some raw sugar and cinnamon; top with ice cream or yogurt.
- Mix ghee and coconut oil; sauté bananas with brown sugar; top with cream or ice cream.

Sauces:

- Ghee is the secret to making perfect Hollandaise Sauce; it's a perfect butter substitute and it's easy to work with.
- Mix ½ cup melted ghee with ½ cup olive oil; refrigerate in container with lid and use for sautéing, spreading, and in sauces calling for olive oil.
- Simmer ghee, white wine, lemon juice, garlic, and a sprig of fresh thyme. Add salt and pour over cooked fish.

Snacks and Appetizers:

- Mix with nut butters such as almond, peanut, cashew and others for an amazing dip for apples and other fruits.

Other Uses:

- Pack it up for traveling, camping, picnicking, and hiking – it's shelf-stable and doesn't need refrigeration.
- Massage into skin instead of lotion or massage oil; it keeps skin and joints supple.
- Keep lips moist: use ghee in place of lip balm.
- Rub ghee into cuticles to help keep nails in good shape.
- Use in place of regular butter for sautéing; it doesn't smoke or burn as easily.
- Use in dairy-free recipes; milk solids are removed from ghee during the clarification process.
- Use in place of vegetable oil for basting, sautéing, and broiling.
- Use in place of butter for drizzling over veggies, pancakes, fish, poultry, and meats.
- Enjoy straight out of the jar!

Notes